America's Health Care System:

What Are The Facts?

ISBN-13: 978-1500209452

ISBN-10: 1500209457

Why is our health care system twice as expensive as those of other countries with poorer outcomes?

This is a continuous real time "book blog" which has tracked daily developments in the American Health Care System for over a year.

This book has an additional digital version which has live links and is continuously updated.

I believe this is a new "forever" book where updates can be read real-time with live links, much like newspapers, except the reader has daily updates and commentary available free of charge over time, after an initial one-time payment.

. The Daily Links and the Daily News

Updated: 2/8/14 The family doctor and drug companies have fueled an explosion in drug overdose deaths? CDC report.
Updated: 2/6/14 What are the facts about the CBO report on Obamacare?
Updated: Are Aging Populations World-Wide Creating Problems?
Updated: 1/29/14 What percent of families have over-weaning medical bills?
Updated: 1/21/14 The Doctor's Lab Coat Can Spread Infection? How?
Updated: 1/18/14 Sepsis Outcomes Seem To Be Unrelated to Hospital Costs
Updated: 1/17/14 Kaiser Former CEO says Hospitals are rewarded for bad care

current plans if they want to?
Updated: 11/13/13 Prescription Related Drug Deaths and Injury at all-time high.
Updated: 11/13/13 Health Care Costs Poised to Take Over the American Economy: New Studies
Updated: 11/12/13 New Study: Health Care Costs Up: Outcomes Down
Updated: 11/12/13 US Official Medicare Website on Medicare and Obama Care Changes
Updated: 11/11/13 Nationwide Update
Updated: 11/10/13 Obamacare and Medicare-- December 7th Deadline.
Updated: 11/7/13 The NPR Take On Obama Care- Cancellations and Subsidies
Updated: 11/6/13 New Ways To Look At Cancer
Updated: 11/6/13 Obamacare and the Cancellations: What Are The Facts?
Updated: 11/4/13 What Social Security Does Not Tell Widowers and Divorcees
Updated: 11/3/13 How Often Do Physicians Disclose the Errors of Other Physicians?
Updated: 10/29/13 Ok, What Are The Facts on Obama Care-For the 15th time.
Updated: 10/28/13 Is Obamacare causing consumers to lose their policies?
Updated: 10/27/13 The End of Antibiotics?
Updated: 10/24/13 What is going on with the Health Care.Gov web site? Hearings.
Updated: 10/21/13 Are There Regional Differences in the kind of care you get?
Updated: 10/17/13 Older person's attitudes toward work and retirement-new study
Updated: 10/27/13 The End of Antibiotics?
Updated: 10/15/13 Hospital CEO pay unrelated to hospital quality and outcomes
Updated: 10/7/13 Dozens of Mental Disorders Don't

Exist At All?
Updated: 10/7/13 Latest study on the costs of Obama Care.
Updated: 10/07/13 What is driving up hospital costs? New study.
Updated: 10/7/13 Hospital Precautions Do Nothing to Stop Infections?
Updated: 10/6/13 Physician Use of Drugs. Is Something to Worry About?
Updated: 10/5/13 Obama Care Depends up Millennials Enrollment
Updated: 10/4/13 The Epidemic in Hospital ICU's
Updated: 9/30/13 Five reasons Americans already love Obama Care-Fox News?
Updated: 9/30/13 Obama Care State By State Costs before Subsidies in a Graph
Updated: 9/30/13 The Battle of the Obama Care Exchanges
Updated: 9/28/13 Obama Care resisted in many Republican States, creating disparities.

Updated: 9/29/13 20 things to know about Obama-Care
Updated: 9/28/13 Senate Health Committee holds hearing on Hospital generated infections and Sepsis-2 hour video
Updated: 9/27/13 Is Congress Exempt from Obama Care?
Updated: 9/27/13 Obama Care Website up and running in time for Oct 1, 2013 enrollment date! Good deal. You can see what it will cost you! Obama Care and Medicare--you can see how it will impact you as well.
Updated: 9/26/13 How Obama Care will affect Medicare?
Updated: 9/26/13 Clinch your jaws, here comes the

government shutdown and debt ceiling battles.
Updated: 9/26/13 The latest report on the costs of Obamacare. The savings are dramatic for most people apparently.
Updated: 9/25/13 Best Websites on Medicare I have found-for you or your parents.
Updated: 9/23/13 Obamacare Oct 1, deadline. What will happen? What you need to know.
Updated: 9/22/13 The Quality of Surgical Care and After Care May be Key to Health and Re-admission rates of Patients
Updated: 9/22/13 Unsafe Medical Care harms 43 million people a year?
Updated: 9/22/13 Antibiotic resistant bacteria: The Danish Example
Updated: 9/19/13 Antibiotic resistant bugs kill 23k a year in the US: CDC-A flurry of reports.
Updated: 9/18/13 Are Anti-biotic resistant deaths down?
Updated: 9/17/13 23 thousand deaths a year in US from infections?
Updated: 9/15/13 New Research on Understanding "What is Health"
Updated: 9/12/13 Do ICU units help patients or not?
Updated: 9/7/13 What is the detail of why American Health Care is so expensive? New Study
Updated: 9/5/13 Kaiser Study finds insurance premiums lower than expected under Obamacare
Updated: 9/5/13 Psychiatry and Drugs. What up with that?
Updated: 9/4/13 The Oct 1st deadline on Obama Care. Are you affected?
Updated: 9/3/13 More data on the costs of Obamacare and who is impacted?
Updated: 8/21/13 How to get fit at any age.
Updated: 8/20/13 Latest Data on the costs of

Obamacare.

how many medical records have errors?
Updated: 6/13/13 Population and the Health Care
System
Updated: 6/8/13 Anti biotic infested meat no longer to
be served in some hospitals. You didn't know?
Updated: 6/4/13 "50 mind-bogging facts about the
American Health Care System?"
Updated: 6/4/13 What are new developments which
might help in treatments to problems identified
above?
Updated: The Bloomberg View of what should be
done about the high health care costs.
Updated: 6/2/13 What the most expensive procedures
in American Health Care?
Updated: 6/1/13 Will Obamacare cause employers to
drop health insurance coverage?
Updated: 5/28/13 Medical Liability, Doctors, Hospitals,
Patients and Medical Outcomes
Updated: 5/27/13 Patient Participation in Health Care
Decison-Making?
Updated: 5/26/13 Ten point check list on what to do
and look for once admission has occurred.
Updated: 5/25/13 Infection rates and death in
hospitals

www.authorsden.com/visit/viewshortstory.asp
Lets explore this question of the quality of our
American Health Care system.

This blog will explore in the coming days several
aspects of the American Health system.

I'll look at cost, mortality rates, infection control, the
hospital incentive structure and other items seeking
an answer to the question to why our health care
system costs twice as much as those of other

countries and we have poor and mediocre outcomes compared to those other countries.

But first we look at the most deadly of all situations for a patient entering a hospital for any reason: the threat of getting infections while there.

This is crucial and hospitals have not solved this problem. Death caused by compilations of surgery, or some other items most often is code for infection and means a patient, even a healthy one, got an infection after being admitted to the hospital. Doctors and hospitals will say pneumonia, sepsis and other seemingly unrelated items or blame it on the age or other unrelated diseases. But shock is a major reaction to serious infections: this leads on to these "complications."
(By the way many surgeons have to redo operations because a sponge was left inside the patient. Sponge counts are critical before closing the patients.)

See:
http://www.sciencedaily.com/releases/2012/12/12121 9111336.htm

We will identify the problem of infection first and then talk about what to do if you or loved one has to go to a hospital-The Wise Patient's Guide to Surviving a Hospital Stay."

See articles on infection below.

http://www.sciencedaily.com/releases/2013/05/13052 2141841.htm

http://www.sciencedaily.com/releases/2013/09/13090

2181001.htm

Private rooms reduce infection and mortality rates

http://www.sciencedaily.com/releases/2011/01/11011
0164742.htm

Patients changing hospitals often carry infections with
them

http://www.sciencedaily.com/releases/2010/03/10031
9085304.htm

Hospitals which cooperate on infection control have
better outcomes

http://www.sciencedaily.com/releases/2012/10/12100
9161059.htm

Infection related deaths in Europe

*http://www.sciencedaily.com/releases/2011/10/11101
1171544.htm*

ICU most dangerous for infections

http://www.sciencedaily.com/releases/2012/10/12101
5161916.htm

What some hospitals are trying in order to control
infections

http://www.sciencedaily.com/releases/2011/08/11081
1181718.htm

A World Wide Study on Infections

http://www.sciencedaily.com/releases/2011/08/11082
4115846.htm

Infections in Nursing Homes

http://www.sciencedaily.com/releases/2010/12/10120
1162115.htm

Putting Grandma in a nursing home can be bad for her health

http://www.sciencedaily.com/releases/2009/06/09060
4095131.htm

Even if you are getting out-patient or in the doctor's office treatments you are not safe

http://www.sciencedaily.com/releases/2009/11/09112
4082801.htm

"MRSA kills an estimated 20,000 people in the United States each year. The superbug, which is resistant to most common antibiotics, can attack wounds and trigger potentially lethal blood stream infections. Community-associated strains, while generally less virulent and susceptible to more antibiotics, can still cause significant morbidity and mortality.

"MRSA has generally been a significant problem only in hospitals," said Eili Klein, the report's lead author and researcher at Resources for the Future. "But the findings from this study suggest that there is a significant reservoir in the community as well." This community reservoir leads to a dangerous spread of community-associated strains from outpatient units into hospitals, according to Klein.

To curtail this spread, hospitals will need to step up infection control procedures, including those practiced in outpatient units."

Medline offers some suggestion on infection control

http://www.nlm.nih.gov/medlineplus/infectioncontrol.html

Over-All National Hospital Rankings for hospitals in the US

First California:
http://www.healthinsight.org/Internal/HospitalPerformanceRankings.html

Now the nation: put your state in the box

http://www.healthinsight.org/Internal/HospitalPerformanceRankings.html

Reducing Healthcare-associated Infections

"99,000 people die due to health care-associated infections (HAI) every year in the United States and nearly **28 to 33 billion dollars are spent** on these infections. Nationwide efforts through many organizations are now working to address this issue.

Healthcare-associated infections

- Put patients at risk
- Increase days of hospitalization
- Add healthcare costs
- Are associated with morbidity/mortality being higher in acute care hospital settings

Are largely preventable (via better hygiene, scientifically tested techniques)"

From:
http://www.healthinsight.org/Internal/Hospital.html

5/26/13

Now we are ready to summarize to this point:
:
1. Infection is important because certain kinds of infections require fluids and/or antibiotics in a matter of hours and others can enter the blood stream and in 24 hours bring on fatal results. So speed is important.

2. Always get the name of the attending doctor and nurse so that you can call and keep up to date from the admission/treatment point from inception.

3. Always ask about what is being used to treat you or a loved one, and what are the alternative, less intrusive options. Never agree to emergency surgery unless you have thoroughly explored the options.

4. Get clear from the beginning on who is making decisions in the family on treatment and at decision points

5. Read up on what complaints or aliments you are dealing with on the internet-before not after treatment.

6. Look up the doctor treating your loved one and the hospital and the department--what has been their infection rates, mortality rates, accreditation issues and the like.

7. Check is to what are the details of any DNR (Do Not *Resuscitate*) you or your loved one might have.

8. If coma is involved ask beforehand if doctors in their treatment plan will induce a comma or not.

Other check lists from attorneys

http://www.urymoskow.com/CM/Articles/10-Things-You-Need-to-Know-About.asp

http://www.bakerandgilchrist.com/legal-services/hospital-malpractice/10-things-you-need-to-know-about-hospitals/

The Consumer Report Hospital Survival Guide
http://www.consumerreports.org/cro/2012/10/your-hospital-survival-guide/index.htm

Sepsis in NY Hospital system. Read this carefully
http://www.nyc.gov/html/hhc/html/safety_quality/prev_inf.shtml

5/27/13
70 percent of patients leave it up to the doctor on health care decisions?

But note doctors and medical law legally assume patients participate and make the decisions-even though we and they know patients don't. Doctors, therefore, have little responsibility if things go wrong. (Same thing is now true in the accounting profession. Audits now mean nothing.)

http://www.consumeraffairs.com/news/studies-examine-the-patients-role-in-healthcare-decision-making-052813.html

 http://www.ct.gov/agingservices/lib/agingservices/pdf/advancedirectivesenglish.pdf

5/28/13

So we ask who exactly is responsible if something goes wrong with treatments from the doctor and the hospital? It varies state by state but let's look at the over-all picture.

First doctors and hospitals have limited their liabilities under various laws such that the burden of proof falls upon the patient, under the guise of "patient rights."

What this actually means is that under most state laws patients are legally responsible for making their own health care decisions, or the family. The doctor is only an "advisor." Couple that with limits on the dollar amounts patients can sue for and limits on class action suits and doctors and hospitals have little liability for patients that die in their care.

15-20 percent of all patients in this country are harmed by the care they received.

If you realize that this occurs with the 2.2 million disease-related deaths a year the number is more than huge.

http://www.cdc.gov/nchs/fastats/deaths.htm

Couple this with the fact that unnecessary testing is done by doctors and hospitals 90 percent of the time on patients resulting in higher hospital and doctor bills as well.

Doctors and hospitals justify all this testing claiming they are protecting themselves from lawsuits, but the fact of the matter is that their incomes are based on tests and procedures they perform and you get at the real reason for the testing-increasing their income.

Moreover, all this testing has been shown to be of little benefit to patients and the picture and incentive structure is clear: more tests, more money for doctors and hospitals. Add infection related income and the picture in not a pretty one.

The argument that such testing reduces doctors and hospitals liability and protects against lawsuits has been shown to be unrelated to both lawsuits and patient outcomes.
What is wrong with this picture?

Let's start with this article:

"However, AHRQ researchers reviewing the impact of these approaches found "little solid evidence" about the impact of medical liability reforms on the cost of care and even less information about the impact of these reforms on patient safety (Hellinger et al.,

2009). Furthermore, the medical liability system may actually hamper progress on patient safety by dissuading physicians from disclosing and examining the root causes of medical errors (Studdert et al., 2004)."

http://www.ahrq.gov/news/newsroom/commentaries/putting-patients-first.html

More info:

http://www.aaos.org/about/papers/position/1118.asp

6/1/13

Will Obama care cause the demise of employer based health care?

6/2/13
What are the specific items which case high costs in the American Health Care System?

http://www.mossadams.com/MA-Perspectives/Will-Employer-Based-Health-Care-Live-or-Die

What are other procedures driving up American health care costs?

"The high price paid for colonoscopies mostly results not from top-notch patient care, according to interviews with health care experts and economists, but from business plans seeking to maximize revenue; haggling between hospitals and insurers that have no relation to the actual costs of performing the procedure; and lobbying, marketing and turf battles among specialists that increase patient fees."

See:

http://www.nytimes.com/2013/06/02/health/colonosco
pies-explain-why-us-leads-the-world-in-health-
expenditures.html?_r=0

http://www.bloomberg.com/news/2013-06-03/the-real-
reason-we-pay-so-much-for-health-care.html

6/4/13

Today we look at new developments in health care
which may, repeat, may, help with some of the issues
identified above.

What are the most promising developments related to
infections and viral diseases?

"We found that the KKL-35 molecule inhibits the
growth of very distantly related bacteria, and this
suggests that it may have antibiotic activity against a
very broad spectrum of species."

As for the Shigella and Bacillus anthracis bacteria,
Keiler said his team was able to show that, "in the
presence of the KKL-35 molecule, these cells died
specifically because the molecule halted the trans-
translation process." Keiler's team also found that,
compared with currently used tuberculosis drug
therapies, the KKL-35 molecule was 100-times more
effective at inhibiting the growth of the strain of
bacteria that causes tuberculosis (Mycobacterium
tuberculosis)."

See:

http://www.sciencedaily.com/releases/2013/06/13060
3163809.htm

New development in suppressing cancer and tumor
suppression:

http://www.sciencedaily.com/releases/2013/06/13060
3163613.htm

New development in treating immune related
diseases:

http://www.sciencedaily.com/releases/2013/06/13060
3133329.htm

But such new developments have many obstacles to
their actual use. Let's explore those tomorrow.

What about cost and the controversy over the actual
costs?

http://www.ncbi.nlm.nih.gov/pmc/articles/PMC263035
1/

Costs, profits and drugs

http://www.slate.com/articles/business/the_customer/
2011/03/the_makebelieve_billion.html

How new drugs are reviewed and approved: A Case
Study

http://www.fda.gov/drugs/developmentapprovalproces
s/howdrugsaredevelopedandapproved/

How do we know that the drug we are taking is the
best and least expensive drug for what ails us? We
don't know.

http://www.amednews.com/article/20121022/professio
n/310229942/4/

Legal and private industry barriers to the use of
generic drugs

http://regulatory.usc.edu/Articles/GenericPharmaceuti
calIndustry.pdf

A summary and really scary view of the American
Health Care System

http://theeconomiccollapseblog.com/archives/50-
signs-that-the-u-s-health-care-system-is-a-gigantic-
money-making-scam-that-is-about-to-collapse

The major cause of bankruptucy in the US is medical
bills which translated means 54 million Americans
cannot afford their high cost medical bills.

http://www.dailymail.co.uk/news/article-2335961/One-
families-pay-medical-bills--meaning-54-million-
Americans-struggle-afford-healthcare.html

True costs of Obama Care?

http://www.washingtonpost.com/blogs/wonkblog/wp/2
013/06/01/the-shocking-truth-about-obamacares-rate-
shock/

6/9/13

Antibiotic infested meat served in some hospitals?
Linked to the superbug?

http://www.nationofchange.org/over-650000-meals-hospitals-will-now-be-served-without-antibiotic-infested-meat-due-super-bugs-13707

6/13/13

Population and the Health Care System

Now we look at a major impactor upon the health care system. Patterns of aging in the US and population growth patterns. First:

http://online.wsj.com/article/SB100014241278873240 49504578541712247829092.html?mod=trending_no w_1

The costs of an aging population rise while the number of working people decline is a formula in both the US and Europe for decline. Populations which do not replicate themselves disappear replaced by immigrants. Similarly, China as the problem stemming from its birth control policy of one child per couple. Russia, Italy and Japan also must be included in this group.

"Perhaps mirroring its declining population growth, European countries tend to have older populations overall. European countries had nine of the top ten highest median ages in national populations in 2005. Only Japan had an older population.[7]"

From:
http://en.wikipedia.org/wiki/Demographics_of_Europe

http://www.indexmundi.com/european_union/populati
on_growth_rate.html

http://epp.eurostat.ec.europa.eu/cache/ITY_OFFPUB/
KS-SF-13-013/EN/KS-SF-13-013-EN.PDF

Also add the fact that technoloy is reducing the
number of jobs, in a technical field like health and the
prospects at first glance look grim.

Let's explore these in the coming days.

6/17/13

Now we look at why hospital costs are so much
higher than doctor costs for the same procedure. And
the issue of medical errors-58% in some cases and
how that can affect your health.

http://mobile.nytimes.com/2013/06/15/health/medicar
e-panel-urges-cuts-to-hospital-payments-for-services-
doctors-offer-for-less.html

"Riddled with errors?

http://m.amednews.com/article/20130617/government
/130619943/1/&template=mobileart

6/17/13

Antibiotics and deaths from infections

http://www.cnn.com/2013/06/13/opinion/boucher-antibiotics-approval/index.html?iid=article_sidebar
Antibiotics given to farm animals related to superbug and infections in the hospital?

http://www.telegraph.co.uk/health/healthnews/10115082/Antibiotics-given-to-farm-animals-could-pose-super-bug-risk-minister-admits.html

"David Willetts, the science minister, said the over-use of antibiotics could be a "big global problem" on the scale of climate change and food security, as bacteria may increasingly grow resistant to the drugs.

Doctors have long been urged to rein in their prescriptions of antibiotics for coughs and colds. However, there are now growing calls for their use to be restricted in agriculture, as superbugs could eventually pass to humans who work on farms or through the food chain."

Education and Health Care

http://opinionator.blogs.nytimes.com/2013/06/16/schooling-ourselves-in-an-unequal-america/

Medical costs and procedures in American Health Care System fail
50% of the time to adequately analyze procedures and methods: new study
http://www.sciencedaily.com/releases/2013/06/130617122236.htm

6/22/13
The Five Most Common Regrets the Dying Have

"A nurse has recorded the most common regrets of the dying, and among the top ones is 'I wish I hadn't worked so hard'. What would your biggest regret be if this was your last day of life?"

http://www.guardian.co.uk/lifeandstyle/2012/feb/01/top-five-regrets-of-the-dying

A nurse has recorded the most common regrets of the dying, and among the top ones is 'I wish I hadn't worked so hard'. What would your biggest regret be if this was your last day of life?

Top five regrets of the dying

A nurse has recorded the most common regrets of the dying, and among the top ones is 'I wish I hadn't worked so hard'. What would your biggest regret be if this was your last day of life?

http://www.guardian.co.uk/lifeandstyle/2012/feb/01/top-five-regrets-of-the-dying

6/20/13

New hope to curtail hospital based infections

http://www.authorsden.com/visit/viewnews.asp?id=41517&authorid=121255
"The paper asserts that one reason for the inefficiency of the U.S. health
care system is its failure to generate and use hard evidence about the
relative benefits of treatment alternatives, such as surgery versus drugs.

Some experts believe that between a third and a half of all U.S. medical
care is not based on or supported by adequate medical evidence.
The lack of evidence raises costs and increases patient risks without
offsetting health benefits, notes the paper," http://www.sciencedaily.com/releases/2013/06/130617122236.htm

http://www.sciencedaily.com/releases/2013/06/130621121003.htm

6/24/13

Breakthroughs in infection fighting
http://www.sciencedaily.com/releases/2013/06/130621121003.htm

http://www.sciencedaily.com/releases/2013/05/130508123024.htm#.UcjW7GS7nxE.email

Hospitals to be fined under Obamacare for re-admissions.

http://www.pbs.org/newshour/rundown/2013/06/hospital-readmissions-a-primer.html

7/4/13

3.2 Million Europeans catch infections every year in hospitals? That is an astounding number

"A survey by the European Centre for Diseases Prevention and Control (ECDC) found that on any given day, one in 18 patients in European hospitals

has at least one hospital-acquired infection -
amounting to around 3.2 million patients per year."

"Worldwide, MRSA infects an estimated 53 million
people annually and costs more than $20 billion a
year to treat. It kills around 20,000 people a year in
the United States and a similar number in Europe."

From:
http://www.reuters.com/article/2013/07/04/us-europe-
hospitals-infections-idUSBRE96309820130704

7/5/13 Antibiotics can harm human tissue?

"Doctors often prescribe antibiotics freely, thinking
that they harm bacteria while leaving human tissue
unscathed. But over the years reports have piled up
about the occasional side effects of various
antibiotics, including tendonitis, inner-ear problems
and hearing loss, diarrhea, impaired kidney function,
and other problems."

From:
http://www.sciencedaily.com/releases/2013/07/13070
3160623.htm

7/8/13

We, in examining the American Health Care System
cannot ignore the prescription drug epidemic the drug
companies have foisted upon American women. Let's
have an initial look.

There is a prescription drug epidemic among women,
landing them in the hospital in record numbers

http://www.alternet.org/drugs/why-it-still-taboo-women-enjoy-taking-drugs?akid=10667.260128.x2u-3f&rd=1&src=newsletter865337&t=8

This article has an oblique point of view but good information is there and the focus is on **hydrocodone.**

7/11/13

Americans living longer but with more health care problems.

"Despite a level of health expenditures that would have seemed unthinkable a generation ago, the health of the US population has improved only gradually and has fallen behind the pace of progress in many other wealthy nations. In fact, by every measure including death rates, life expectancy, and diminished function and quality of life as assessed by the authors, the US standing compared with 34 Organization for Economic Co-operation and Development countries declined between 1990 and 2010."

http://www.cinemablend.com/pop/Americans-Living-Longer-With-More-Health-Problems-57411.html

http://online.wsj.com/article/SB10001424127887324694904578597444105321914.html#project%3DHEALTH20130710%26articleTabs%3Dinteractive

http://www.usatoday.com/story/news/nation/2013/07/10/age-mental-decline/2505371/

http://www.reuters.com/article/2013/07/10/us-usa-health-studies-idUSBRE96901320130710

7/12/13

http://www.google.com/hostednews/afp/article/ALeqM5gWejXWbjGjheZNu1DHK_TDjQl5YQ?docId=CNG.7bbff7de88b7143a6295e17894a259aa.191

http://www.wate.com/story/22807017/us-lagging-other-countries-on-many-health-measures?clienttype=mobile

7/14/13

http://www.sciencedaily.com/releases/2012/05/120514153111.htm

7/21/13

How widespread are errors and misdiagnosis in American Health Care

http://www.sciencedaily.com/releases/2013/07/130719085154.htm

http://www.sciencedaily.com/releases/2013/04/130422211747.htm

http://www.sciencedaily.com/releases/2011/02/110207225947.htm

7/23/13

Race and Health Care Outcomes

http://www.sciencedaily.com/releases/2011/10/111006173614.htm

 http://www.sciencedaily.com/releases/2010/03/100315125555.htm

http://www.sciencedaily.com/releases/2008/10/081020171231.htm

http://www.sciencedaily.com/releases/2010/04/100428110814.htm

Which is safer, cities or rural areas

http://www.latimes.com/news/science/sciencenow/la-sci-sn-safer-in-the-city-20130723,0,3803327.story

http://usnews.nbcnews.com/_news/2013/07/23/19623252-surprise-big-cities-safer-than-small-towns-study-finds

7/26/13
35 things you need to know about 911, ER treatments and ambulances

http://www.rd.com/health/wellness/35-more-secrets-the-er-staff-wont-tell-you/

7/31/13

You or a loved one needs surgery. What are the Consumer Reports Ratings for hospitals in the United States?

8/2/13

Obama Care: What are the facts:
#Last, but certainly not least - premium changes are unlikely to affect you at all. The rates submitted to states and the federal governments are for coverage sold to individuals and small businesses with fewer than 50 workers that are not self-insured. Currently, the vast majority of Americans with insurance coverage get it through their jobs – and they generally work for companies with more than 50 workers. Large firms already offer coverage similar to what the health law will require insurers to offer individuals and small firms, so little change is expected. The new rates are most likely to affect people who buy their own coverage. About 15 million do so currently and an estimated 7 million more are expected to do so next year because of the health law.

From:
http://www.webmd.com/health-insurance/20130801/five-things-to-know-about-obamacare-premiums-a-guide-for-the-perplexed?page=2

8/3/13

Trillions of dollars spent. Who or what is getting all that money?

http://healthland.time.com/2013/02/20/what-makes-health-care-so-expensive/

8/18/13

The Deadly Truth About Sepsis. What you need to know

http://www.google.com/gwt/x?u=http://www.aarp.org/health/conditions-treatments/info-08-2013/sepsis-what-you-need-to-know.html&ei=7IkLUtX2F8OvkQLu6oDYCA&wsc=pb

http://www.google.com/gwt/x?wsc=pb&u=http://healthtools.aarp.org/health/sepsis&ei=f4oSUusU4o-QApTMgbgl

The deadly truth is that this can kill you even when you are already in a hospital, but they miss the diagnosis and you get an infection from the hospital itself. See above in this blog for more information about Sepsis which I consider to be one of the most deadly of all diseases, because it can kill you in 48 hours. So speed of treatment is essential, especially if you are in a foreign country.

Quote:

"Sepsis is a life-threatening condition that arises when the body's response to infection causes system-wide inflammation, injuring tissues and organs. It's sometimes called blood poisoning, and a number of cases occur as a result of seemingly benign incidents — like a scrape on the playground or even a large paper cut.

In other cases, like Kerri's, sepsis can start out as a garden-variety infection but quickly turn into something more serious. Frighteningly, the number of people hospitalized for sepsis has more than doubled in the past decade, partly due to increasing antibiotic resistance as well as an aging population.

"Every week I have to tell three or four families that their loved ones are dying from something most of them have never heard of," says intensive care physician Jim O'Brien, M.D., of Riverside Methodist Hospital in Columbus, Ohio. Sepsis strikes seemingly at random, and sometimes is missed even by seasoned physicians. "We don't have a diagnostic test for sepsis. And doctors have not organized our care around sepsis like we have around

From:
http://www.google.com/gwt/x?u=http://www.aarp.org/health/conditions-treatments/info-08-2013/sepsis-what-you-need-to-know.html&ei=7IkLUtX2F8OvkQLu6oDYCA&wsc=pb

8/20/13
Latest Data On the Cost of Obamacare?

http://www.latimes.com/business/la-fi-insurance-costs-20130821,0,807175.story

8/21/13
How to get Fit At Any Age?

http://www.cnn.com/2013/08/20/health/fitness-any-age/?hpt=he_c1

9/3/13
Who is impacted by Obamacare?

http://www.pbs.org/newshour/rundown/2013/09/how-will-the-obamacare-mandate-impact-you.html

9/4/13
Oct 1st and Obama Care. Are you affected?

http://www.businessweek.com/articles/2013-09-03/what-small-businesses-need-to-do-for-obamacare-before-oct-dot-1#r=read

9/5/13 Psychiatry and Drugs. What is up with that?

http://www.newyorker.com/online/blogs/elements/2013/09/psychiatry-prozac-ssri-mental-health-theory-discredited.html?mbid=gnep&google_editors_picks=true

9/5/13
Kaiser Study finds insurance premiums lower than expected under Obamacare

http://thehill.com/blogs/healthwatch/health-reform-implementation/320369-group-finds-lower-than-expected-obamacare-premiums-in-broad-study

9/7/13

Why is US health care so expensive?

http://healthland.time.com/2013/02/20/what-makes-health-care-so-expensive/

http://healthland.time.com/2013/02/20/what-makes-health-care-so-expensive/?utm_source=buffer&utm_campaign=Buffer&utm_content=buffer7782a&utm_medium=twitter

9/12/13
Do ICU help or do they merely provide expensive futile care?

http://www.pentagonpost.com/15-icu-patients-may-be-getting-futile-treatment-survey/83411830

9/15/13
New Research on Understanding "What is Health?"

"We often think of human cells as tiny computers that perform assigned tasks, where disease is a result of a malfunction. But in the current issue of *Science*, researchers at The Mount Sinai Medical Center offer a radical view of health -- seeing it more as a cooperative state among cells, while they see disease as result of cells at war that fight with each other for domination."

From:

http://www.sciencedaily.com/releases/2013/09/130912143217.htm

Help with Sepsis

http://www.sciencedaily.com/releases/2013/09/130912143215.htm

9/17/13

http://www.nytimes.com/2013/09/17/health/cdc-report-finds-23000-deaths-a-year-from-antibiotic-resistant-infections.html?_r=0

9/18/13
Are Anti-biotic resistant deaths down?

http://www.medpagetoday.com/InfectiousDisease/GeneralInfectiousDisease/41656

http://www.motherjones.com/tom-philpott/2013/09/cdc-meat-industry-yes-you-contribute-antibiotic-resistance

9/19/13
http://rt.com/usa/drug-resistant-bacteria-us-979/

http://www.motherjones.com/tom-philpott/2013/09/cdc-meat-industry-yes-you-contribute-antibiotic-resistance

http://www.medicalnewstoday.com/articles/266182.php

http://www.bloomberg.com/news/2013-09-16/gonorrhea-among-drug-resisting-germs-sickening-millions.html

http://www.nbcnews.com/health/animals-repeatedly-infected-people-mers-study-suggests-4B11203299

http://minnesota.publicradio.org/display/web/2013/09/16/health/antibiotic-resistant-microbes

9/22/13
Antibiotic resistant bacteria: The Danish Example

"In 2012, 1,556 Danes were found positive with methicillin-resistant staphylococci -- MRSA. This represents an increase of 20% from 2011. In fact, the total number of cases has almost doubled since 2009. MRSA bacteria are resistant to antimicrobial agents that are essential for treatment of treating life-threatening infections in humans."

From:
http://www.sciencedaily.com/releases/2013/09/13091
9085436.htm

9/22/13
Unsafe Medical Care harms 43 million people a year?

'More than 43 million people are injured worldwide each year due to unsafe medical care, according to a new study from Harvard School of Public Health (HSPH). These injuries result in the loss of nearly 23 million years of "healthy" life."

From:

http://www.sciencedaily.com/releases/2013/09/13091
8211617.htm

9/22/13

The Quality of Surgical Care and After Care May be Key to Health and Re-admission rates of Patients

"The results showed that approximately one in seven patients discharged was readmitted within 30 days.

Hospitals with the best performance on two well-established measures of hospital surgical quality, surgical volume and 30-day mortality rates, had much lower readmission rates than other hospitals. For example, hospitals in the highest quartile for surgical volume had a significantly lower readmission rate than hospitals in the lowest quartile (12.7% vs. 16.8%). Hospitals with the lowest surgical mortality rates had a significantly lower readmission rate than hospitals with the highest mortality rates (13.3% vs. 14.2%)."

From:

http://www.sciencedaily.com/releases/2013/09/130918180417.htm

9/23/13
Obamacare Oct 1, deadline. What will happen? What you need to know.

http://www.nytimes.com/2013/09/23/health/lower-health-insurance-premiums-to-come-at-cost-of-fewer-choices.html?pagewanted=all&_r=0

9/25/13

Best Websites on Medicare and Medicaid I have found-for you or your parents.

The official Medicare Web site

http://www.medicare.gov/

http://www.medicare.gov/sign-up-change-plans/

http://www.socialsecurity.gov/pubs/EN-05-10043.pdf

Social Security Mistakes Not to Make

http://www.pbs.org/newshour/businessdesk/2013/09/the-danger-of-trusting-social.html

"In these 36 states, a single 27-year-old would pay an average of $214 a month for the lowest-cost silver plan before the tax credit. After the credit is applied, it would cost $145 a month, which is an additional 33 percent discount. The federal government would pay the difference of $69 a month directly to the insurer, which, is a boon for their business but also saves that 27-year-old $828 a year in out-of-pocket expenses."

From:
http://www.alternet.org/personal-health/obamacare-costs-lower-tax-subsidies-higher-expected?akid=10976.260128.cR_YYZ&rd=1&src=newsletter901448&t=5

See also on the deficit and the debt ceiling battle

http://www.washingtonpost.com/blogs/wonkblog/wp/2013/09/26/the-falling-deficit-has-been-a-disaster-for-the-gop/

More on Obama Care

"Just 27 percent of people ages 19 to 29 had heard of the health insurance exchange marketplaces, where people who don't get coverage at work will be able to shop for insurance plans and learn whether they qualify for subsidized benefits, the Commonwealth Fund poll of almost 1,900 people between November 2011 and March 2013 reveals. Awareness was even lower among people who were uninsured during part of the prior year and whose incomes will make them eligible for help, at 19 percent and 18 percent, respectively."

From:
http://www.huffingtonpost.com/2013/08/21/young-adults-obamacare_n_3786805.html

More:

http://blog.aarp.org/2013/09/25/new-health-plan-premiums-will-be-less-than-expected/

How will Obama Care affect Medicare?

http://www.pbs.org/newshour/bb/health/july-dec13/health_09-26.html

9/27/13
Obama Care Website is up and running in time for Oct 1, 2013 enrollment date! Good deal. You can see what it will cost you!

https://www.healthcare.gov/

Obama Care and Medicare. How will it affect you?

http://obamacarefacts.com/obamacare-medicare.php

For those who like a Q and A session: See video

http://www.democracynow.org/

Is Congress exempt from Obama Care

http://www.usatoday.com/story/news/politics/2013/09/27/is-congress-exempt-from-obamacare/2883635/

9/28/13

Senate Health Committee holds hearing on Hospital Generated Infections and Sepsis-2 hour video

http://www.c-span.org/Events/Efforts-to-Reduce-Healthcare-Associated-Infections/10737441634-1/

What is the situation in Europe?
http://www.sciencedaily.com/releases/2011/10/111011171544.htm

9/28/13

Obama Care resisted in many Republican States, creating disparities.

http://www.washingtonpost.com/opinions/how-obamacare-could-create-new-health-disparities/2013/09/27/5994cdd8-248f-11e3-b75d-5b7f66349852_story_1.html

9/29/13

20 things to know about Obama-Care- Pretty good list

http://starbeacon.com/nationalnews/x1836123258/20-things-to-know-about-the-Affordable-Care-Act

9/30/13

The battle of the Obama Care exchanges

 http://mobile.reuters.com/article/idUSBRE98R0A220130929?irpc=932

 http://www.politico.com/story/2013/09/as-shutdown-looms-obamacare-exchanges-still-set-for-launch-97510.html?hp=t3_3

 http://www.nytimes.com/news/affordable-care-act/2013/09/30/survey-shows-confusion-over-health-care-law-but-support-for-medicaid-expansion/?_r=0

9/30/13

Five reasons Americans already love Obama Care
    http://www.foxnews.com/opinion/2013/09/30/five-reasons-americans-already-love-obamacare-plus-one-reason-why-theyre-gonna/

10/4/13
The Epidemic in Hospital ICU's

 http://www.sciencedaily.com/releases/2013/10/131002185238.htm

 http://www.sciencedaily.com/releases/2013/05/130514212946.htm

 http://www.sciencedaily.com/releases/2012/12/121207094325.htm

10/5/13
Obama Care Depends upon Millennials Enrollment

http://www.cbsnews.com/8301-18563_162-57606214/obamacares-success-rests-on-attracting-uninsured-millennials/

10/6/13
Physician Use of Drugs. Is Something to Worry About?

http://www.sciencedaily.com/releases/2013/10/131004124937.htm

Prostate Cancer Testing: Useful or Useless?

http://www.sciencedaily.com/releases/2013/10/131004090817.htm

10/7/13
Hospital Precautions Do Nothing to Stop Infections?

http://guardianlv.com/2013/10/study-hospital-precautions-do-nothing-to-stop-infections/

10/07/13
What is driving up hospital costs. New study.

http://www.sciencedaily.com/releases/2013/10/131002125518.htm

10/7/13
Latest study on the costs of Obama Care.

http://www.sciencedaily.com/releases/2013/10/13100
1151130.htm

10/7/13

Dozens of Mental Disorders Don't Exist At All?
http://life.nationalpost.com/2013/10/07/dozens-of-
mental-disorders-dont-exist-and-dsm-5-is-a-fiction-of-
ideology-u-s-therapist-claims-ahead-of-world-mental-
health-day/

Updated: 10/15/13

Hospital CEO pay unrelated to hospital quality and
outcomes

http://www.reuters.com/article/2013/10/14/us-hospital-
quality-care-idUSBRE99D0MA20131014

10/17/13
Older person's attitudes toward work and retirement-
new study

http://www.sciencedaily.com/releases/2013/10/13101
5103941.htm

10/21/13
Are There Regional Differences in the Kind of Care
You Get? What are the variations between hospitals
merely a few miles apart?

http://www.latimes.com/opinion/commentary/la-oe-
1015-welch-too-much-medicine-
20131015,0,5854399.story

"In the late 1980s, both the Lancet and the New England Journal of Medicine published the findings that Boston residents were hospitalized 60% more often than their counterparts in New Haven. Oh, by the way, the rate of death — and the age of death — in the two cities were the same."

10/24/13

Health Care.Gov website. What is going on? Hearings

http://www.pbs.org/newshour/rundown/2013/10/watch-live-testimony-on-healthcaregov-problems.html

10/27/13
The End of Antibiotics?

http://www.upi.com/Health_News/2013/10/27/Expert-The-end-of-antibiotics-period/UPI-59881382932519/

10/28/13

Is Obamacare causing consumers to lose their policies?

"By all accounts, the new policies will offer consumers better coverage, in some cases, for comparable cost -- especially after the inclusion of federal subsidies for those who qualify. The law requires policies sold in the individual market to cover 10 "essential" benefits, such as prescription drugs, mental health treatment and maternity care. In addition, insurers cannot reject people with medical problems or charge them higher prices. The policies must also cap consumers' annual expenses at levels lower than many plans sold before the new rules."

From:
http://www.pbs.org/newshour/rundown/2013/10/why-the-health-reform-law-is-causing-thousands-to-lose-coverage.html

10/29/13

Ok, What Are The Facts on Obama Care-For the 15th time?

 http://touch.latimes.com/#section/-1/article/p2p-77973264/

11/3/13

How Often Do Physicians Disclose the Errors of Other Physicians?

 http://www.sciencedaily.com/releases/2013/10/131030185712.htm

 http://www.nytimes.com/2013/11/04/business/under-health-care-act-millions-eligible-for-free-policies.html?_r=0

11/4/13
What Social Security Does Not Tell Widowers and Divorcees

http://www.pbs.org/newshour/businessdesk/2013/11/how-social-security-keeps-divorces-and-widows-in-the-dark-about-their-benefits.html

 11/6/13
Obama Care and the insurance company cancellations: What Are The Facts?

http://www.motherjones.com/mojo/2013/11/obamacare-repeal-cancellation-notice

http://www.motherjones.com/kevin-drum/2013/11/obamacare-will-be-boon-millions-people

New Ways To Look At Cancer
www.nydailynews.com/life-style/health/daily-news-guide-medicare-part-ii-glossary-key-terms-article-1.1512518

http://www.motherjones.com/environment/2013/10/inquiring-minds-george-johnson-cancer-myths-reality

11/7/13
The NPR Take On Obamacare

http://www.npr.org/blogs/health/2013/11/07/243584170/how-the-affordable-care-act-pays-for-insurance-subsidies?sc=tw

11/10/13

Obamacare and Medicare--December 7th Deadline.

http://www.nydailynews.com/life-style/health/daily-news-guide-medicare-part-ii-medigap-plans-article-1.1512508

Impact on Supplemental Plans
http://www.nydailynews.com/life-style/health/guide-medicare-open-enrollment-ends-dec-7-article-1.1512498

Definition of Terms

http://www.nydailynews.com/life-style/health/daily-news-guide-medicare-part-ii-glossary-key-terms-article-1.1512518

11/11/13

http://www.nbcnews.com/health/dont-expect-big-enrollment-numbers-health-insurance-exchanges-2D11577708

11/12/13

US Official Medicare Website on Medicare and Obama Care Changes
http://www.medicaresolutions.com/pdf/MedicareAndYou2014.pdf

http://www.nydailynews.com/life-style/health/guide-medicare-open-enrollment-fine-tune-part-best-drug-prices-article-1.1477949

http://www.medicaresolutions.com/planlistmedicare.aspx

11/12/13

New Study: Health Care Costs Up: Outcomes Down

http://www.businessweek.com/news/2013-11-12/health-improvements-in-u-dot-s-dot-slow-even-as-costs-rise-study-finds http://health.usnews.com/health-news/news/articles/2013/11/12/soaring-prices-not-demand-behind-massive-hike-in-us-health-spending

11/13/13

"New estimates released from the Office of the Actuary at the Centers for Medicare and Medicaid Services (CMS) project that aggregate health care spending in the United States will grow at an average annual rate of 5.8 percent for 2012-22, or 1.0 percentage point faster than the expected growth in the gross domestic product (GDP)"

From:
http://www.sciencedaily.com/releases/2013/10/131010091704.htm

http://www.sciencedaily.com/releases/2013/11/131112095336.htm

11/13/13

Prescription drug and Injury related deaths at an all-time high in the US

http://www.sciencedaily.com/releases/2013/11/131112003432.htm

http://www.sciencedaily.com/releases/2011/03/110301122144.htm

http://www.sciencedaily.com/releases/2012/10/121015131545.htm

http://www.sciencedaily.com/releases/2010/11/10110
1161829.htm

11/16/13

Obamacare: How good is the President's promise that
everyone can keep their current plans if they want to?

http://www.theatlantic.com/business/archive/2013/11/
everything-you-need-to-know-about-obamas-new-
you-can-keep-your-plan-policy/281522/

 NPR audio on Obama care and keeping your current
health plan.

http://www.npr.org/blogs/health/2013/11/15/24547321
1/will-you-get-to-keep-your-health-plan-depends-on-
where-you-live?sc=tw

 http://www.npr.org/blogs/health/2013/11/15/2454212
24/consumer-guide-to-obamas-plan-for-canceled-
health-policies?sc=tw

11/17/13

Obamacare: How Will It Affect Supplemental Plans
and Medicare Advantage Plans?

http://www.lasvegassun.com/news/2013/nov/17/us-
on-the-money-medicare-advantage/

11/17/13

The Crisis of Antibiotics.

http://abcnews.go.com/Health/wireStory/drug-resistant-bacteria-spreading-europe-20903051

https://news.google.com/news/section?pz=1&cf=all&topic=m&siidp=83e8e9766e48c33ffb467c672d45351a5cf2&ict=ln

11/18/13

Obesity and Antibiotic use. A state by state study

http://www.motherjones.com/environment/2013/11/maps-antibiotics-prescriptions-obesity-states

11/18/13

Early signs of a heart attack early. What are they?

http://www.nbcnews.com/health/signs-sudden-heart-attack-may-appear-month-study-suggests-2D11624552

Today's Generation is less fit?

http://children.webmd.com/news/20131119/kids-worldwide-getting-less-heart-fit-research-shows

11/20/13

Is Health Care Spending Down Sharply Due to Obamacare?

http://www.usatoday.com/story/news/nation-now/2013/11/20/health-care-spending-growth/3650243/

11/22/13

The Poor Die of Treatable Diseases, Why? A Doctor's Report
http://www.alternet.org/i-watched-my-patients-die-treatable-diseases-because-they-were-poor?paging=off&current_page=1#bookmark

11/25/13

New Method to diagnose Sepsis. Could save thousands of lives

http://www.sciencedaily.com/releases/2013/11/131119082927.htm

11/26/13
Obamacare allows single-payer?

http://m.dailykos.com/story/2013/11/24/1258135/-Obama-just-launched-single-payer-in-America

11/29/13
Is Health Care Spending Down Sharply Since Obamacare?

http://www.nytimes.com/2013/11/29/opinion/krugman-obamacares-secret-success.html?_r=0

12/3/13
http://www.pbs.org/newshour/rundown/2013/12/the-medical-service-you-havent-heard-of-could-save-hospitals-billions.html

12/3/13
Extra stiches cost 500 dollars?
http://www.nytimes.com/2013/12/03/health/as-hospital-costs-soar-single-stitch-tops-500.html

12/3/13
Hospital Costs: Do They Make Any Sense?

http://www.sfgate.com/business/bottomline/article/Convoluted-hospital-pricing-under-scrutiny-5032279.php

12/8/13
Are Drug Trials Sponsored by the Drug Industry Biased? Duh.

http://www.sciencedaily.com/releases/2010/08/100802173713.htm

12/10/13

What you need to know when the hospital or ER tells you will be held for "observation."

http://health.yahoo.net/articles/healthcare/observation-status-what-it-means-hospitals-and-patients

12/10/13
The expensive and wildly varying cost of ambulance rides.

http://priceonomics.com/the-wild-west-of-ambulance-charges/

12/11/13
Physician Crisis?

http://www.healthcarefinancenews.com/news/crisis-physician-recruitment?topic=,,24

1/6/14

Do Hospitals Have a Financial Incentive to Pull the Plug on Your Loved One? The Case of Jahi McMath

http://www.sfgate.com/opinion/openforum/article/Hospital-incentive-to-bury-mistakes-must-be-5115986.php

1/10/14

Smoking what are the numbers?

"43: percent of Americans who smoked in 1964

18: percent of Americans who smoke today

7,000: the number of scientific studies the U.S. surgeon general's advisory committee examined before declaring that smoking caused lung cancer, laryngeal cancer and chronic bronchitis

17.7 million: the number of Americans who died from tobacco-related causes between 1964 and 2012. (A chain-smoking doctor among Terry's expert report authors was diagnosed with lung cancer within a year of the surgeon general's announcement, NPR reports. He later died of the disease.)

8 million: the estimated number of tobacco-related deaths in the U.S. that anti-smoking initiatives have prevented since 1964

19.6: The average numbers of year's people add to their lifespans by not smoking regularly"

From:

http://www.popsci.com/article/science/100-years-smoking-studies-popular-sciencewww.popsci.com/article/science/100-years-smoking-studies-popular-science

`1/13/14

How the Mediterranean Diet can save your life.

http://www.alternet.org/personal-health/big-pharmas-best-kept-secret-mediterranean-diet-can-save-your-life?akid=11398.260128.dWxrai&rd=1&src=newsletter946302&t=18

1/13/14 Big Agriculture's Role in the Antibiotic Disaster

"There is a near consensus among public health experts that the bulk antibiotics produced by AHI's member companies are accelerating the approach of a post-antibiotics nightmare scenario, in which superbugs routinely emerge from our farms and wreak havoc on a human population living among the ruins of modern medicine."

From:

http://www.alternet.org/food/factory-farms-are-accelerating-antibiotics-

nightmare?akid=11398.260128.dWxrai&rd=1&src=ne
wsletter946302&t=14

1/17/14

Former Kaiser CEO says hospitals are rewarded for
bad care.

http://www.pbs.org/newshour/bb/health/jan-
june14/health_01-17.html

1/18/14

High-Cost Hospitals Do Not Have Higher Sepsis
Survival Rates

http://www.sciencedaily.com/releases/2011/02/11022
8163032.htm

1/21/14

"Studies have shown doctors' clothing may spread
infectious diseases to patients.

New recommendations have been issued to help
prevent possible contamination."

Read more:
http://www.wptv.com/dpp/news/health/doctors-white-
coats-may-spread-infectious-diseases-to-patients-
study-says#ixzz2r4A8Eh48

1/29/14

Medical bills and the American Family

http://www.latimes.com/science/sciencenow/la-sci-sn-medical-costs-burden-on-families-20140128,0,7524866.story#axzz2roLF6lom

2/2/14

Are Aging Population Creating Problems World Wide?

http://www.usatoday.com/story/news/nation/2014/01/30/world-population-aging-america/5044447/

 2/6/14

What does the CBO report really say about Obamacare, job killer or good news?

See video report below

http://www.democracynow.org/2014/2/6/job_killer_how_media_spin_got

 "Summarized Kessler: "Thus, some people might decide to work part-time, not full-time, in order to keep getting health-care subsidies. Thus, they are reducing their supply of labor to the market. Other people near retirement age might decide they no longer need to hold onto their job just because it provides health insurance, and they also leave the work force.

"Look at it this way: If someone says they decided to leave their job for personal reasons, most people would not say they 'lost' their jobs. They simply decided not to work," he said."

From:
 http://www.deseretnews.com/article/865595684/CBO -report-Workers-may-reduce-hours-under-health- care-law.html

 For sticklers: Here is an actual copy of the report.

http://www.cbo.gov/sites/default/files/cbofiles/attachm ents/45010-Outlook2014.pdf

 2/8/14

Do whatever you can but don't let your loved ones get hooked on legal and prescription drugs.
Oxycontin is basically heroin and just as difficult to kick.

"Between 2000 and 2010 the number of people that died from drug overdoses more than doubled from 17,000 to 38,000, according to the most recent figures from the Centers for Disease Control and Prevention.

In 2009, for the first time in US history, more people died from drugs overdoses than from traffic accidents or firearms, although that is partly because the numbers of gun deaths and road deaths are both decreasing. So what is causing this epidemic?

The data suggests the number of people overdosing from pharmaceutical - or prescription - drugs has trebled over that decade, just as the quantity of prescription painkillers sold to pharmacies, hospitals, and doctors' offices has quadrupled over the same period."

From:

http://www.bbc.co.uk/news/magazine-26067987

See part two of this blog at:

http://www.authorsden.com/visit/viewshortstory.asp?id=60454&authorid=121255

6/10/14 Red Meat Linked to Breast Cancer?
6/2/14 What day and what time you get surgery may affect death rate in hospitals?
6/2/14 Revolutionary Treatment in Hard To Cure Cancers?
6/1/14 Two or more slices of white bread are bad for you?
5/31/14 The 1,000 dollar pill. Big battle starting between insurance companies and drug companies
5/24/14 New discovery in the fight against infection
5/11/14 New guidelines on hospital associated infections: diarrhea.
5/8/14 Hospitals Doing Too Many C Sections? Why? New Consumer Report
5/2/14 The most deadly animal
5/2/14 The Antibiotic Time Bomb
5/2/14 CDC report: 40 percent of deaths has just five causes
5/2/14 The Antibiotic Crisis: Bigger Than the Aids Crisis? CDC Report
4/20/14 Doctors hate their jobs and 300 commit

suicide each year? Why?

4/9/14 Who determines the prices we pay for Medicare?

4/14 Drug company scams?

4/9/14 Put in your doctors name find out how much he/she gets in Medicare payments and for what.

4/6/14 Off the shelf stick-on health monitoring? Looks Like it.

4/1/14 Republicans Going After Medicare Again at; http://www.nbcnews.com/politics/first-read/what-ryans-budget-means-doesnt-mean-medicare-n69011

4/1/14

Occupancy rates above 92 percent means increased mortality rates. new study says yes.

"Hospital Occupancy Rates Above 92 percent results in higher mortality rates? New Study says Yes at: The paper's authors attribute the effect to the fact that the number of personnel hospitals assign to their wards is only sufficient to cope with average levels of occupancy. If the occupancy tipping point is consistently exceeded, the result is a persistent safety problem and failure to appropriately adjust the number of personnel may lead to a significantly increased threat to the survival of hospitalized patients."

From:
http://www.sciencedaily.com/releases/2014/03/14033 1100234.htm

4/1/14 Republicans Going After Medicare Again
Updated: 3/26/14 Who Decides How Much Your

Medical Bills Will Be and How?
Updated: 3/26/14 1 in 25 patients with hospital associated infections- CDC Study
Updated: 3/23/14 Cause of Sepsis Identified?
Updated: 3/13/13 Key Finding in How to Prevent Heart Failures
Updated: 3/11/14 One Social Security Mistake NOT to make.
Updated: 3/2/14 All about anti-depressants. The News is Not Good.
Updated: 2/27/14 A Doctors Stethoscope Can Carry Germs? Apparently
Updated: 2/25/14 Acetaminophen linked to ADHD in Children.
Updated: 2/25/14 Medicare: Inpatient vs. Observation: Thousands of Dollars At Stake.
Updated: 2/24/14 National Rankings of US Hospitals. Where is yours?
Updated: 2/24/14 Many Medicare Patients Get Pain Killers From Multiple Doctors
Updated: 2/21/14 New Budget From White House cuts Medicare 2 percent.
Updated: 2/20/14 Obama Drops Plan to Cut Social Security Benefits
Updated: 2/18/14 How many parents and in what states are parents not having their kids vaccinated?
Updated: 2/13/14 Medicare Advantage Plans to be Cut? Who wins and who loses?

4/1/14 Republicans Going After Medicare Again at;

http://www.nbcnews.com/politics/first-read/what-ryans-budget-means-doesnt-mean-medicare-n69011

http://www.nytimes.com/2014/04/02/us/politics/paul-ryan-budget.html?hpw&rref=politics

http://www.politico.com/story/2014/04/paul-ryan-budget-medicare-health-care-105234.html

2/13/14
Medicare Advantage Plans: Who Wins and Who Loses?

Senior Benefits At Risk?

http://www.washingtonpost.com/national/health-science/doctors-cut-from-medicare-advantage-networks-struggle-with-what-to-tell-patients/2014/01/25/541bfbd8-77b4-11e3-af7f-13bf0e9965f6_story.html

2/18/14

How many parents and in what states are parents not having their kids vaccinated?

http://www.motherjones.com/environment/2014/02/vaccine-exemptions-states-pertussis-map?google_editors_picks=true

2/20/14

Obama Drops Plan to Reduce Social Security

Good, Mr. President.

http://thehill.com/blogs/on-the-money/budget/198815-obama-abandons-cut-to-social-security

2/21/14

White House Cuts Medicare 2%

https://mail.google.com/mail/u/0/h/1kf3gz5savq69/?&v=c&th=14456c36d34bc416

2/24/14

http://thecelebritycafe.com/feature/2014/02/high-number-medicare-patients-are-getting-painkillers-multiple-doctors

2/24/14

National Hospital Rankings.

http://healthinsight.org/rankings/hospitals

2/25/14

Medicare: Whether you are admitted as "Inpatient" or "Under Observation"

It could mean thousands of dollars in costs for you.

http://www.nbcnews.com/video/nightly-news/54026469/#54026469

2/25/14

Acetaminophen linked to ADHD in children of mother who took the drug which is in many drugs, most over the counter. Hundreds of drugs use it.

http://www.knowyourdose.org/common-medications

http://www.wbay.com/story/24818139/2014/02/25/study-acetaminophen-tied-to-risk-of-adhd

http://www.reuters.com/article/2014/02/25/us-prenatal-acetaminophen-idUSBREA1O1UO20140225

2/27/14
A doctor's stethoscope can carry germs. Maybe?

http://www.philly.com/philly/health/topics/HealthDay685307_20140227_Doctors__Germ-Laden_Stethoscope_May_Spread_Nasty_Bacteria.html

3/2/14

All about anti-depressants. The News is Not Good.

http://www.sciencedaily.com/releases/2014/02/140225122429.htm

http://www.sciencedaily.com/releases/2011/07/110719121354.htm

http://www.sciencedaily.com/releases/2010/11/101122111510.htm

3/11/14

One Social Security Mistake Not to Make

http://www.pbs.org/newshour/making-sense/one-call-social-security-doom-financial-future/

3/13/14

Key Discovery in how to prevent heart failure?

"Subsequently, the researchers at the Cardiovascular Research Center at Icahn School of Medicine at Mount Sinai found that injecting a small piece of RNA to inhibit the effects of miR-25 dramatically halted heart failure progression in mice. In addition, it also improved their cardiac function and survival."

http://www.sciencedaily.com/releases/2014/03/140312150101.htm

3/23/14 Cause of Sepsis Identified?

http://www.sciencedaily.com/releases/2014/03/140321094859.htm

3/26/14

1 in 25 hospital patients acquire hospital associated infections. 243 thousand deaths

http://thegazette.com/2014/03/26/cdc-1-in-25-patients-contracts-an-infection-during-hospital-stay/

3/26/14

http://truth-out.org/news/item/22693-of-patients-and-prices

4/6/14

http://www.sciencedaily.com/releases/2014/04/140403212615.htm

http://www.washingtonpost.com/business/economy/data-uncover-nations-top-medicare-billers/2014/04/08/9101a77e-bf39-11e3-b574-f8748871856a_story.html

Put in your doctors name- find out how much he gets in Medicare payments

http://www.washingtonpost.com/wp-srv/special/national/medicare-doctors-database/

http://www.washingtonpost.com/business/economy/an-effective-eye-drug-is-available-for-50-but-many-doctors-choose-a-2000-alternative/2013/12/07/1a96628e-55e7-11e3-8304-caf30787c0a9_story.html

Medicare prices

http://www.washingtonpost.com/business/economy/medicare-pricing-drives-high-health-care-costs/2013/12/31/24befa46-7248-11e3-8b3f-b1666705ca3b_story.html

4/20/14

"You don't train someone for all of those years in [medicine]... and then have them run a claims processing operation for insurance companies."

http://www.thedailybeast.com/articles/2014/04/14/how-being-a-doctor-became-the-most-miserable-profession.html

5/2/14

The Antibiotic Crisis: Bigger Than the Aids Crisis? CDC Report

http://www.timeslive.co.za/Feeds/2014/05/02/antibiotic-crisis-bigger-than-aids

http://www.dw.de/antibiotic-resistant-germs-a-bacterial-time-bomb/a-17606199

The most deadly animal

http://www.businessinsider.com/bill-gates-mind-blowing-infographic-mosquiotes-2014-4#!HmAoq

5/8/14

Hospitals Doing Too Many C Sections? Why? New Consumer Report

http://www.nydailynews.com/life-style/health/hospitals-performing-c-sections-reports-article-1.1785129

5/11/14
Source of many hospital associated infections

http://www.sciencedaily.com/releases/2014/05/140506120236.htm

5/24/14
New Hope in the fight against bacteria resistant infection?

http://www.sciencedaily.com/releases/2014/05/140522175719.htm

5/31/14

The 1,000 dollar pill. Big battle starting between insurance companies and drug companies

http://thehill.com/policy/healthcare/206797-insurance-lobby-lets-beat-government-to-drug-cost-reform

6/1/14

Two or more slices of white bread per day is bad for you?

http://m.timesofindia.com/Home/Science/White-bread-consumption-linked-to-obesity/articleshow/35810207.cms

6/2/14

Revolution in hard to cure cancers?

http://www.houstonchronicle.com/news/health/article/Revolution-in-cancer-treatment-reported-5523437.php http://www.cbsnews.com/news/immune-therapy-shows-promise-against-cervical-cancer/

6/2/14
Surgery days and time may affect mortality rates in hospitals?

http://news.health.com/2014/06/02/does-timing-play-a-role-in-survival-after-hospital-admission-surgery/

6/10/14

Red Meat Linked to Breast Cancer?

http://www.kansascity.com/living/article518142/Study-Red-meat-possibly-linked-to-breast-cancer.html

END